THE ACENE

(The Acne Cure And
Maintainers) Just Another
Four Letter Words

I0480831

Success Israel

Table of Contents

CHAPTER ONE

INTRODUCTION

Acne: is a pores and skin situation that happens while your hair follicles end up plugged with oil and useless pores and skin cells. It reasons whiteheads, blackheads or zits. Acne is maximum not unusual place amongst teenagers, eleven though it influences human beings of every age.

Effective pimples remedies are available, however pimples may be persistent. The zits and bumps heal slowly, and while one starts to head away, others appear to crop up. Depending on its severity, pimples can reason emotional misery and scar the pores and skin. The in advance you begin remedy, the decrease your chance of such troubles.

SYMPTOMS

Acne symptoms and symptoms range relying at the severity of your situation:

· Whiteheads (closed plugged pores) · Blackheads (open plugged pores) · Small pink, soft bumps (papules) · Pimples (pustules), that are papules with pus at their tips · Large, solid, painful lumps beneathneath the pores and skin (nodules) · Painful, pus-stuffed lumps beneathneath the pores and skin (cystic lesions)

Acne generally seems at the face, forehead, chest, top lower back and shoulders. When to peer a health practitioner If self-care treatments do not clean your pimples, see your number one care health practitioner. He or she will be able to prescribe more potent medicines. If pimples persists or is excessive, you could need to are trying to find clinical remedy from a health practitioner who specializes within side the pores and skin (dermatologist or pediatric dermatologist).

For many girls, pimples can persist for decades, with flares not unusual place every week earlier than menstruation. This kind of pimples has a tendency to remedy without remedy in girls who use contraceptives.

In older adults, a surprising onset of excessive pimples can also additionally sign an underlying sickness requiring clinical attention.

The Food and Drug Administration (FDA) warns that a few famous nonprescription pimples creams, cleansers and different pores and skin merchandise can reason a severe response. This kind of response is pretty rare, so do not confuse it with any redness, inflammation or itchiness that happens in regions wherein you have implemented medicines or merchandise.

Seek emergency clinical assist if after the use of a pores and skin product you revel in:

· Faintness · Difficulty breathing · Swelling of the eyes, face, lips or tongue ·

CAUSES

Four important elements reason pimples:

· Excess oil (sebum) manufacturing · Hair follicles clogged through oil and useless pores and skin cells · Bacteria · Inflammation

Acne usually seems in your face, forehead, chest, top lower back and shoulders due to the fact those regions of pores and skin have the maximum oil (sebaceous) glands. Hair follicles are related to grease glands.

The follicle wall can also additionally bulge and convey a whitehead. Or the plug can be open to the floor and darken, inflicting a blackhead. A blackhead can also additionally appear like dust caught in pores. But truly the pore is congested with micro organism and oil, which turns brown while it is uncovered to the air.

Pimples are raised pink spots with a white middle that broaden while blocked hair follicles end up infected or inflamed with micro organism. Blockages and irritation deep interior hair follicles produce cyst like lumps below the floor of your pores and skin. Other pores for your pores and skin, that are the openings of the sweat glands, are not generally worried in pimples.

Certain matters can also additionally cause or get worse pimples:

· Hormonal adjustments. Androgens are hormones that growth in boys and ladies throughout puberty and reason the sebaceous glands to increase and make extra sebum. Hormone adjustments throughout midlife, especially in girls, can result in breakouts too. · Certain medicines. Examples encompass pills containing corticosteroids, testosterone or lithium. · Diet. Studies imply that ingesting positive meals — consisting of carbohydrate-wealthy meals, consisting of bread, bagels and chips — can also additionally get worse pimples.

Further take a look at is wanted to have a look at whether or not human beings with pimples could gain from following precise nutritional restrictions. ·

Stress. Stress does not reason pimples, however when you have pimples already, strain can also additionally make it worse.

CHAPTER TWO

ACNE MYTHS

These elements have little impact on pimples:

·   Chocolate and greasy meals. Eating chocolate or greasy meals has little to no impact on pimples. ·   Hygiene. Acne is not as a result of grimy pores and skin. In fact, scrubbing the pores and skin too difficult or cleaning with harsh soaps or chemical substances irritates the pores and skin and may make pimples worse. ·   Cosmetics. Cosmetics do not always get worse pimples, in particular in case you use oil-loose make-up that does not clog pores (noncomedogenics) and put off make-up frequently. Nonoil cosmetics do not intrude with the effectiveness of pimples pills.

Beings with lighter pores and skin to revel in those pimples complications:

·   Scars. Pitted pores and skin (pimples scars) and thick scars (colloids) can continue to be long-time period after pimples has healed.   ·   Skin adjustments. After pimples have cleared, the affected pores and skin can be darker (hyper pigmented) or lighter (hypo pigmented) than earlier than the situation occurred.

Risk elements

Risk elements for pimples encompass:

· Age. People of every age can get pimples, however it is maximum not unusual place in teenagers. · Hormonal adjustments. Such adjustments are not unusual place throughout puberty or pregnancy. · Family history. Genetics performs a function in pimples. If each of your mother and father had pimples, you are probable to broaden it too. · Greasy or oily substances. You can also additionally broaden pimples wherein your pores and skin comes into touch with oil or oily creams and lotions. · Friction or strain in your pores and skin. This may be as a result of objects consisting of telephones, cell phones, helmets, tight collars and backpacks.

What are the signs of pimples?

Acne may be observed nearly everywhere in your frame. It maximum generally develops in your face, lower back, neck, chest, and shoulders.

If you've got pimples, you'll usually be aware zits which can be white or black. Both blackheads and whiteheads a re called comedowns.

Blackheads open on the floor of your pores and skin, giving them a black look due to oxygen within side the air. Whiteheads are closed simply beneathneath the floor of your pores and skin, giving them a white look.

While whiteheads and blackheads are the maximum not unusual

place lesions visible in pimples, different kinds also can arise. Inflammatory lesions are much more likely to reason scarring of your pores and skin. These encompass:

- Papules are small, pink, raised bumps as a result of infected or inflamed hair follicles.
- Pustules are small pink zits which have pus at their tips.
- Nodules are solid, frequently painful lumps below the floor of your pores and skin.
- Cysts are big lumps observed below your pores and skin

that comprise pus and are
generally painful.

CHAPTER TREE

Acne happens while the pores of your pores and skin end up blocked with oil, useless pores and skin, or micro organism.

Each pore of your pores and skin is the outlet to a follicle. The follicle is made from a hair and a sebaceous (oil) gland.

The oil gland releases sebum (oil), which travels up the hair, out of the pore, and onto your pores and skin. The sebum maintains your pores and skin lubricated and soft.

One or extra troubles on this lubrication technique can reason pimples. It can arise while:

- an excessive amount of oil is produced through your follicles
- useless pores and skin cells acquire for your pores
- micro organism increase for your pores

These troubles make a contribution to the improvement of zits. A pimple seems while micro organism grows in a clogged pore and the oil is not able to escape.

What are the chance elements for growing pimples?

Myths approximately what contributes to pimples are pretty not unusual place. Many human beings trust that meals consisting of chocolate or French fries will make a contribution to pimples. While there's no medical assist for those claims, there are positive chance elements for growing pimples. These encompass:

- hormonal adjustments as a result of puberty or pregnancy
- positive medicines, consisting of positive

delivery manipulate capsules or corticosteroids

- a weight loss plan excessive in subtle sugars or carbohydrates, consisting of bread and chips
- having mother and father who had pimples

People are maximum at chance for growing pimples throughout puberty. During this time, your frame undergoes hormonal adjustments. These adjustments can cause oil manufacturing, main to an accelerated chance of pimples. Hormonal pimples associated with puberty generally subsides, or as a minimum improves whilst you attain adulthood.

How is pimples diagnosed?

If you've got signs of pimples, your health practitioner could make a prognosis through inspecting your pores and skin. Your health practitioner will pick out the forms of lesions and their severity to decide the quality remedy.

How is pimples dealt with?

At-domestic care

There are some self-care sports you could attempt at domestic to save you zits and remedy your pimples. Home treatments for pimples encompass:

- cleansing your pores and skin day by day with a slight cleaning soap to put off extra oil and dust
- shampooing your hair frequently and preserving it from your face
- the use of make-up that's water-primarily based totally or labeled "noncomedogenic" (now no longer pore-clogging)

- now no longer squeezing or choosing zits, which spreads micro organism and extra oil
- now no longer carrying hats or tight headbands
- now no longer touching your face.

CHAPTER FOUR

MEDICATION

If self-care doesn't assist together along with your pimples, some over the counter pimples medicines are available. Most of those medicines comprise elements that may assist kill micro organism or lessen oil in your pores and skin. These encompass:

- Benzyl peroxide is found in many pimples lotions and gels. It's used for drying out current zits and stopping new ones. Benzyl peroxide additionally kills pimples-inflicting micro organism.

- Sulfur is a herbal element with a specific odor that's observed in a few creams, cleansers, and masks.

- Resorcinol is a much less not unusual place element used to put off useless pores and skin cells.

- Salicylic acid is frequently utilized in soaps and pimples washes. It allows save you pores from getting plugged.

Sometimes, you could retain to revel in signs. If this happens, you could need to are trying to find clinical advice. Your health practitioner can prescribe medicines that could assist lessen your signs and save you scarring. These encompass:

- Oral or topical antibiotics lessen irritation and kill the micro organism that reason zits. Typically, antibiotics are simplest used for a quick time in order that your frame doesn't increase a resistance and depart you at risk of infections.
- Prescription topical lotions consisting of retinoic acid or prescription-electricity

benzyl peroxide is frequently more potent than over the counter remedies.

- Pimples thru a lower in oil manufacturing.

Isotretinoin (Acutance) is a vitamin-A-primarily based totally medicine used to deal with positive instances of excessive nodular pimples. It can reason severe aspect effects, and it's simplest used while different remedies don't paintings.

Your health practitioner can also additionally advocate approaches to deal with excessive pimples and save you scarring. These:

- to lessen oil manufacturing and micro organism. Other lasers can be used by myself to assist enhance pimples or scarring.

- gets rid of the pinnacle layers of your pores and skin with a rotating brush and could be quality for treating pimples scarring in place of a remedy for pimples. Microdermabrasion is a milder remedy that allows put off useless pores and skin cells.

- A chemical peel gets rid of the pinnacle layers of your pores and skin. That pores and skin peels off to expose much less broken pores and skin underneath. Chemical peels can enhance slight pimples scarring.

- Your health practitioner can also additionally recommend the use of cortisone injections in case your pimples includes big cysts. Cortisone is a steroid certainly produced through your frame. It can lessen irritation and velocity healing. Cortisone is generally used along side different pimples remedies.

What is the outlook for a person with pimples?

Treatment for pimples is frequently successful. Most human beings can assume their pimples to start clearing up inside six to 8 weeks. However, flare-ups are not unusual place and might require extra or long-time period remedy. Isotretinoin is the remedy maximum probable to offer everlasting or long-time period nice results.

Acne scarring can reason emotional misery. But, set off remedy can assist save you scarring. Also, your dermatologist could have remedy alternatives designed to deal with scarring.

HOW CAN PIMPLES BE PREVENTED?

It's hard to save you pimples. But you could take steps at domestic to assist save you pimples after remedy. These steps encompass:

- washing your face two times an afternoon with an oil-loose cleanser
- the use of an over the counter pimples cream to put off extra oil
- warding off make-up that includes oil

- casting off make-up and cleansing your pores and skin very well earlier than bed
- showering after exercising
- warding off tight-becoming clothing
- ingesting a healthful weight loss plan with minimum subtle sugars
- lowering strain

Speak together along with your health practitioner to research extra approximately techniques to manipulate your pimples.

THE END